NATURAL HEALTH
HANDBOOK

NATURAL HEALTH HANDBOOK

Seven Ways to Wellness

Teresa Gregurek

To order additional copies of this book, contact:
Xlibris Corporation
1-888-795-4274
www.Xlibris.com
Orders@Xlibris.com

My goal for this book is to teach others some of the basic ideas I have learned in the past 13 years as a natural health consultant. Most of the information in this book is what I teach others in small groups. I wanted a way to reach many more people than I could through my business – Herbs To Go. This book is an independent publication and has not been funded or assisted by any supplement manufacturer. I am an independent distributor and Manager with Nature's Sunshine Products and I do mention specific products listed in Bold print throughout the book. These are available thru my website – www.herbstogo.com.

The information in this book is for educational and personal use and is not meant to diagnose or treat disease. You should see a competent health practitioner for any serious medical condition.

CONTENTS

WATER

Your body needs good pure water to maintain health, to keep organs working, and to remove toxins. Symptoms of not getting enough water include constipation, poor digestion, and dry skin, among others. A guide to how much water to drink is to take your weight in pounds, divide by half, and drink that many ounces of water daily (example – wt. of 150 lbs divided by half = 75, so drink 75 oz daily). Coffee, soda, tea, and other beverages don't count. Some of these act as diuretics and actually remove water from your body. Coffee is acidic for your body. Drink purified water, not tap water containing chlorine and chemicals. Buying a water purifier is more affordable than bottled water and also better for the environment. Remember – if you don't filter your water, your kidneys and liver have to filter it. You need these organs to function for a healthy life. The costs for kidney dialysis and liver transplants are enormous.

It is better to take sips of water throughout the day than to drink four ounces or more at one time. Drinking sips allows your cells to absorb more and won't keep you in the bathroom as much. If you don't like the taste of plain water, squeeze in some fresh lemon juice (this lemon water helps to alkalize the body and also helps to prevent or soften kidney stones). **Liquid Chlorophyll** can also be added to your water. This gives a mint taste, helps to get rid of any body odors such as smelly feet, helps your body cool off in hot weather, acts as a detoxifier and helps bring oxygen to the body.

Drinking adequate water also helps your digestion. It is best to avoid drinking more than four ounces of liquids with your meals. Too much liquid in the stomach dilutes the enzymes needed to digest your food and can lead to indigestion and reflux. Drink water when you get up in the morning and between meals. The structural system needs water to provide fluid around your joints. Dehydration can lead to more joint pain.

Water is very important for elimination of wastes by the body. It helps to prevent constipation if you drink the recommended amount of water daily. Optimally, you should have a bowel movement for every meal you eat (example – if you eat 3 meals per day, you should eliminate 3 times or 2 times at minimum). If this isn't working with your diet, add an extra fiber supplement (**Psyllium Hulls Combo, Loclo, Nature's Three, Everybody's Fiber**, and/or a natural herbal laxative such as **Gentle Move** or **LBS**). If you are not eliminating wastes, toxins can build up in the intestines. By eliminating adequately, you will also have a flatter abdomen. Colon transit times can be measured to determine adequate elimination. To do this, you can eat beets or corn, and then look at your stools when you have bowel movements over the next few days. About 24 hours is considered good transit time. (If you see evidence in your stool of the corn or beets (red color) within 12 hours, this could mean you are eliminating too fast and may not be absorbing nutrients adequately. If it takes 36 hours or more, you could have sluggish elimination and this could lead to toxins being stored in your intestines.

The water you use to shower or bathe in should be filtered also. Inexpensive shower filters can be purchased. Most city water supply contains chlorine and other chemicals – these are absorbed into your skin and into your lungs when you shower. Daily use over years can lead to toxin build-up in the body. You will notice the difference in your hair and skin when you use a filter for your shower.

PH BALANCE

pH is a measure of the acidity or alkalinity of a solution. The lower the number – the more acidic the solution. The higher the number, the more alkaline the solution. You can use pH test strips to check the pH of your urine and saliva. The goal is to keep your ph within the 6-7 range for optimal health. Maintaining optimum pH helps with energy levels, digestion, cardiovascular & structural health, immunity, and ideal weight. Proper pH also allows minerals to be absorbed by the body from the food you eat and supplements you take. Iodine is the mineral that has the narrowest range (6.3-6.6) for it to be absorbed. This mineral is important for thyroid function and metabolism; if it isn't absorbed it may interfere with weight loss. Foods that help the body become more alkaline include asparagus, broccoli, lemons, limes, watermelon, and grapefruit. Foods that are most acidic include white flour, pasta, pork, beef, shellfish, cheese, milk, beer, and soft drinks. Also acidic are many artificial sweeteners such as NutraSweet, Equal, and Sweet N'Low. There are many foods in between. A goal is to try to eat 80% alkaline foods and 20% acidic foods for a balanced pH.

Supplements to help an acidic body achieve balanced pH include **magnesium, liquid chlorophyll**, and **food enzymes**. Use **Rose Hips** or **Citrus Bioflavonoids** if you take Vitamin C, instead of **Vitamin C with ascorbic acid**. Supplements to help an alkaline body become pH balanced include **Milk Thistle** (to aid in liver detoxification), **flax seed oil**, **Vitamin C Timed Release, food enzymes, liquid calcium**.

Try a detox bath to balance pH – use 1 cup Epsom salts, 1 cup baking soda, 2 tsp. **ginger** (can use 10 capsules **ginger**-open up the capsules, mix all ingredients together). Add these to a bathtub of hot water, soak for 20 minutes, then rinse off, doing this 2-3 times per week.

Stress also affects your body's pH. Stress usually causes too much acidity in the body. Find ways to help relieve stress (exercise, music, doing something you enjoy, being outside in nature, etc.). Practice and learn how to do deep breathing exercises – this will help to provide more oxygen to the body and relieve stress and balance pH. **Lavender** essential oil is very calming and helps with stress and insomnia (rub on or spray on feet at night).

Disease cannot grow in a balanced ph.

DIET

The amount and types of supplements you take will not help if you continue to eat an unhealthy diet. Keep a food diary for 2 weeks with everything you eat each day and how you felt that day. This will help you learn which foods you may be allergic to, or which types of foods you may be eating incorrectly, for your individual body. (Feeling sleepy during the day might mean you ate too many carbohydrates and not enough protein). A guide to use to see how much protein your body needs is to multiply your body weight in pounds by 0.37 (this would equal grams of protein/day needed). Besides beef, chicken, and fish, good protein sources also include eggs, nuts, protein shakes, beans (pinto, black beans, lentils, chickpeas, and hummus). Protein meal replacement shakes include **Nutri-Burn**, **Love and Peas**, **SmartMeal,** and **Nature's Harvest**.

Carbohydrates include simple carbs and complex carbs. Simple carbs are foods which make blood sugar go up quickly such as white flour, white sugar, pastries, and fruits – especially fruit juices. Complex carbohydrates include brown rice, whole grain breads – these don't cause blood sugar to go up as quickly. Low glycemic vegetables and fruits also help prevent spikes in blood sugar. These include zucchini squash, broccoli, green beans, cabbage, leafy salad greens, apples, cherries, grapefruit, and pears. High glycemic vegetables and fruits can cause blood sugar to rise rapidly. These include white potatoes, corn, pineapple, grapes, melons, bananas, oranges, and orange juice. There are glycemic lists of foods available to help guide you in your choices. A goal is to keep your blood sugar stable throughout the day to avoid cravings, snacking, and fatigue.

There are good fats and bad fats. Good fats improve your cholesterol levels, reduce your risk of heart disease, help you feel full, and may help you lose weight. Good sources of fats include olive oil, fish, avocados, and nuts (walnuts, pecans, almonds, and macadamias). Bad fats include hydrogenated oils and transfats (read labels on products to see what is included). These bad fats lead to inflammation in the body which causes many chronic diseases. It is better to avoid processed foods since these often contain bad fats, additives, and preservatives. Your body needs the good fats for brain and nervous system function and for production of hormones. If you supply your body with bad fats, your cells will reproduce with these, leading to a chain reaction causing damage to your DNA, which can lead to heart disease and tumor growth.

The Blood Type Diet comes from research published in the two books by Dr. Peter D'Adamo. This involves knowing your particular blood type (O, A, B, or AB) and following the diet as to the foods which are beneficial for you and knowing what foods to avoid. Benefits of this are reported to be more energy, less illness, better digestion, fewer allergies, and weight loss.

A guide to use for the number of calories needed to maintain your weight is to multiply your body weight x 10 (example – 150 lbs x 10 = 1500 calories). A recent research study involving thousands of people showed none of them received the RDA (recommended daily allowance) of vitamins and minerals needed from their diet, so a daily multivitamin/mineral is essential. **Super Supplemental** is a good choice. Also, once you are over 35 years old, there is a decrease in enzymes produced in your stomach to digest food. Raw food (fresh fruits and vegetables, not cooked) contain enzymes, but when foods are cooked, the enzymes are destroyed. **Food**

Enzymes should be taken with meals when you are eating cooked foods.

It is very important to eat some form of protein within the first hour of awakening in the morning. This will start your metabolism and help your energy level throughout the day. Never skip breakfast. **Spirulina** is a supplement that can be taken in capsule form which is a source of protein, as well as Vitamin B12. It can be carried with you to take for those times when you might have to go too long between meals.

It is best to avoid artificial sweeteners – these go by names such as Splenda, Sucralose, Aspartame, Nutra-Sweet. Ingesting these adds chemicals to your body and research has shown these have been linked to causing joint pain, mood swings, migraine headaches, fatigue, nervous system problems, bloating and diarrhea. Safer alternatives are natural sweeteners including stevia and xylitol, which have very few calories and do not affect your blood sugar. Other natural sweeteners include honey, agave, and maple syrup – although these can affect blood sugar and diabetics should use them only in small amounts. Splenda (sucralose) is made by adding chlorine to sugar. Aspartame converts to methanol when heated above 86 degrees, in the body during digestion, it is converted to formaldehyde. Some of these also destroy the good bacteria in your intestines.

Find alternatives to soft drinks. The phosphoric acid upsets the body's calcium phosphorus ratio, weakens bones contributing to osteoporosis, and also can contribute to kidney stone formation.

The sugar or corn syrup in soft drinks contributes to a major cause of obesity.

Avoidance of MSG (monosodium glutamate) is also very important. This is considered to be an excitotoxin – damaging to the nervous system. It is often on labels by other names, especially if the label lists many artificial ingredients and preservatives. Taking **Vitamin E with Selenium** counteracts the effects of MSG. MSG can cause migraine headaches, mood swings, and depression. Research has shown this substance added to food made lab animals eat more food to the point they became obese. Read labels and try to avoid or limit your processed food intake.

Xenoestrogens are false estrogens. These are found in meats (chicken, beef), and eggs in which the animals were given hormones. They trick the body into thinking they are true hormones and can cause hormonal imbalance, early puberty in children, breast enlargement, etc. Organic meats and eggs do not have these xenoestrogens. Many plastics also contain these toxins which can leach out and get into foods (if it is heated in the microwave – for example). Do not leave plastic water bottles out in the sun and then later drink out of them – the sun can break down the plastic and cause these to get in the water. Xenoestrogens are also found in pesticides and many home cleaning products.

Using a microwave to heat food is not a good choice. This changes the composition of the food and can have many long term effects. Never stand close to a microwave while it is on (there is an electromagnetic field – EMF, around it). Do your own research on this – look this up on www.mercola.com and read more about this. There are other ways to heat food quickly such as convection ovens, etc.

IMMUNE SYSTEM PROTECTION

Your body's immune system helps to protect against foreign substances such as bacteria, viruses, etc. At least 60-70% of your body's immunity comes from the intestinal system. This is through the friendly bacteria in your gut. Antibiotics destroy many of these good bacteria. To increase the friendly bacteria, have a stronger immune system, and decrease your incidence of colds, flu, viruses, "food poisoning" etc., you can eat foods that supply the good bacteria or take Probiotic supplements. Cultured foods with good bacteria include sauerkraut, natural live yogurt – without sugar and preservatives, kefir, kimchee. Probiotic supplements include **Acidophilus, Bifidophilus**, and **Probiotic Eleven**. Take probiotic supplements on an empty stomach, such as first thing in the morning when you awaken, or at night before bedtime.

Washing your hands frequently helps to prevent the spread of germs and resulting illness. It is better not to use antibacterial hand soaps since these destroy the natural acid-mantle skin protection, and bacteria can also become resistant to these. There are many natural and chemical free soaps which can be used. (Your skin absorbs anything you put on it, so minimizing chemicals puts less load on the liver to detoxify and causes less allergic reactions). On a personal note, women who use tampons during a menstrual period should know many of these products are bleached with chlorine or dioxins, which can disrupt hormones. (Buy organic all cotton tampons).

Eating a well balanced diet and avoiding or minimizing sugar and junk food can help your immune system. Eating sugar depresses your immune system for 4 hours. Sugar also increases growth of cancer cells in the body. Most soft drinks contain 1 tsp. sugar/ounce.

Vitamin/Herbal products for the Immune system include **Silver Shield, Thai-Go, Olive Leaf, Echinacea, Garlic, Elderberry D3fense, Vitamin C**, and others. When taking **Vitamin C** in large doses – take to bowel tolerance (when you start having loose stools, decrease the dose). **Silver Shield w/AquaSol** is a patented product which is very safe to use. Research has shown that between 90-99 percent of this is excreted by the body by the next day, so there is no toxic accumulation in the body compared with the older "colloidal" silver products. (Silver has been used since ancient times – by the Romans for storing water, wine, and vinegar; by the doctors in the early 1800's for silver sutures to stitch wounds; and was used to sterilize recycled water in the space vehicles by the former Soviet Union). This **Silver Shield with Aqua Sol** formula is effective in destroying many dangerous bacteria such as salmonella, E.coli, Pseudomonas aeruginosa and Streptococcus, as well as the resistant staph bacteria (MRSA). It is also effective against many viruses by making them unable to replicate, or reproduce. **Silver Shield** is a product to have on hand in your home first aid supply. It has been recommended as a safe resource in the area of bioterrorism by the U.S. government director of Integrative Center for Homeland Security. (It is also available in gel form for topical use and can be used for wounds and as a hand sanitizer, plus many other uses). **Thai-Go** is a juice drink which is a concentrated form of very high antioxidants including mangosteen fruit, blueberries, raspberries, green tea, apple extract, red grapes, acai berry, pomegranate, red grapeseed extract, plus more. It provides immune support to the body by helping to get rid of "free radicals" which are caused by environmental pollutants among other things. The ingredients also help the circulatory system and work against any inflammation in the body. (Most chronic diseases are caused by inflammation). **Thai-Go** has been tested by an independent commercial lab (Brunswick Labs), and rated the highest on an antioxidant scale compared with several other top-selling antioxidant drinks on the market today. The recommended daily amount to drink is 2 ounces/day for a maintenance daily supplement. **Olive leaf extract** is a standardized concentrate in capsule form which provides antibacterial and circulatory system support, and is effective against many bacteria, viruses, and fungus. **Echinacea** is an herb that can help strengthen the immune system; it is available in capsule or liquid form, it has been known as a blood purifier, and is often used for respiratory infections. **Elderberry D3fense** is an herbal formula in capsule form which contains elderberry, Echinacea, Vitamin D3, and royal jelly. Elderberry has been shown in research to prevent replication of the flu virus in the body – effective against 8 strains of the flu. **Vitamin D3** (the sunshine vitamin) is synthesized in the body with the help of sunshine. During the winter months, it may be hard to be outside to get any sunshine, depending on where you live. Most of us are deficient in this vitamin, based on lab tests done. Research has shown low Vitamin D levels cause increased risk of breast cancer, diabetes in children, infertility, arthritis progression, SAD (seasonal affective disorder), obesity, influenza, and childhood tooth decay – if the mother was deficient during pregnancy. Royal jelly is made by worker bees and fed to the queen bee; it has antimicrobial and healing properties and contains many nutrients.

Get enough sleep (7-9 hours/night) to allow your immune system to repair. Your body repairs itself during sleep. Sleep deprivation can lead to altered blood sugar metabolism and contributes to diabetes. It can also speed the aging process and lead to obesity.

In cases of eating "bad food " or " food poisoning", **Activated Charcoal** capsules can be taken by mouth to absorb toxins (capsules can also be opened and put in water to drink). **Aloe vera juice** also helps to relieve intestinal distress. **Roman chamomile essential oil** mixed with **massage oil** can be rubbed on the abdomen to relieve cramps and intestinal spasms. **Cramp Relief** capsules can be taken also to help. **Peppermint essential oil** can help nausea – just by smelling the oil. It can also be rubbed on abdomen with massage oil.

Essential oils to help the immune system include **Guardian blend, Wild Oregano, & Eucalyptus**, among others. These should never be applied directly on the skin. Use a carrier oil such as **massage oil** or **aloe vera gel** or even olive oil, if nothing else available. These can be rubbed on the soles of the feet, or mixed in a bath or foot soak, or also be put in a diffuser to help respiratory problems, by having the essential oils in the air in a room. **Oregano oil** is very strong, only use a few drops in a foot bath (it has been known to get rid of a cold, if used when symptoms first begin). Essential oils are absorbed through the skin in seconds and act as antibacterial, antifungal, and antiviral agents. Always use high quality essential oils which come from the true plant or flower. Synthetic oils can cause allergic reactions and also will not give you true healing results.

Other ways to help your immune system would be to limit exposure to electromagnetic fields (EMF). Do not put your cell phone next to your bed or under your pillow when you sleep – at least put it in the next room. Limit your cell phone use – use texting or use landline phones whenever you can. Having a lot of EMF exposure at night can interfere with your sleep – it can disrupt your brain's production of melatonin. To find out more about EMF, look up Dr. Mercola's website.

If you are having problems with respiratory allergies, try eating a small amount of local honey on a daily basis (honey produced by bees within the area where you live, within 50 miles). This could help your body adjust to the pollen in your area. **Histablock** is an herbal formula which helps with hayfever type symptoms. **ALJ** is another herbal formula which helps support the respiratory system and helps to get rid of mucous; it contains horseradish.

All body cells regenerate within a period of 7 years, so you can have an entire new body in 7 years, if you work on your health with nutrition and supplements. (Skin cells get replaced quickly, blood cells take about 4 months, and bone takes 7 years). Hering's Law of Cure says the body heals itself from the mind down, from inside out, and in reverse order of symptoms suppressed.

EXERCISE

Find an activity you enjoy that you can do 3-5 times per week at minimum. This helps you maintain or lose weight, increases your immunity, helps your mood, and relieves stress. A mini-trampoline can be used to help move lymphatic fluid in your body – this acts as a detoxifier. Start slow when using a trampoline, no more than 5 minutes on first few days, and then gradually increase the time on it. (Going too long at first can move too many toxins in the body and you may feel ill).

Supplements to help with exercise: **Herbal Trim Skin treatment** can be applied to the skin before exercise and acts as a body wrap (spa treatment). You can add **Cellu-Tone essential oil** to this to help shrink cellulite. **Tei Fu Massage lotion, MSM/Glucosamine Cream**, or **Everflex Pain cream** can be used for sore muscles or joints after strenuous exercise.

Solstic Revive is an instant beverage mix in stick pack form which you add to 16 oz. bottle of water, to drink as a natural electrolyte replacement drink. **Solstic Energy** is another instant beverage that has a small natural source of caffeine, no sugar, B vitamins, and green tea.

CoQ10 helps to provide energy to the heart muscle and to all your cells. It is normally present in your body but decreases as you age. It is also decreased if you are on statin drugs (to lower cholesterol). **Target Endurance Formula** provides energy and endurance during exercise. **Energ-V** contains bee pollen and other herbs to provide energy.

DETOX

There are many forms and ways to remove toxins from your body. Doing a cleanse usually gives you more energy, may eliminate or reduce allergy symptoms, can help you lose weight, slows aging, and offers many other benefits. It is recommended to do a cleanse 2 times/year, usually in spring and fall. Toxins are stored in fat cells. When an overweight person tries to lose weight too quickly, this may result in toxins being released and feeling ill. An obese person may have difficulty losing weight due to the body's protective effect of not wanting to release the toxins.

Those who should not do a cleanse include pregnant or nursing women, weak, emaciated, or extremely fatigued individuals.

Detox baths can be used by mixing 1 cup Epsom salts, 1 cup baking soda, and 2 tsp. ginger (or about 10 capsules ginger opened up and mixed with the Epsom salts and baking soda). Add to bathtub of hot water, soak for 20 minutes, then rinse off, may do this 2-3 times/ week. Bentonite is a form of clay that pulls out toxins; this can be used in a bath (1 cup), use 2 times per month. This is available as **Hydrated Bentonite**.

Your body's organs of elimination include the skin, colon, kidneys, and lungs. If any of these organs are blocked, you may have problems with one of the other sites of elimination.

Signs of toxins in the colon could include constipation, swelling of the abdomen, bad breath, poor digestion, food allergy, weight issues, and poor energy. Herbal formulas for the colon include **Clean Start, Liquid Cleanse**, and **Tiao He Cleanse**.

Signs of toxins in the kidneys include kidney stones, lower backaches, frequent urination, knee and leg cramps, water retention, and joint weakness. Herbal formulas for the kidneys to help cleanse include **Cranberry Buchu, Chinese Kidney Activator**, and **Kidney Drainage**. Freshly squeezed lemon juice in water can be taken to help soften kidney stones. Black cherry juice can also help kidney problems.

Signs of toxins in the lungs include coughing and congestion, various lung ailments, arm weakness, poor posture, and inadequate breathing. Herbal formulas for the lungs include **ALJ,** and **Chinese Breathe EZ**.

Signs of toxins in the skin include rashes, cysts, and poor skin color. Herbal formulas for the skin include **Ayurvedic Skin Detox, Chinese Liver Balance**, and **Lymph Gland Cleanse**.

All Cell Detox is an overall body detox formula. Research has shown impaired detoxification is linked to many diseases such as cancer, chronic fatigue, fibromyalgia, and Parkinson's disease. **Enviro-Detox** is another formula which acts as a blood purifier and has immune system support.

Symptoms indicating a need for a liver cleanse include feelings of anger, bitterness, mood swings, etc. It is very important to do an intestinal cleanse first to make sure you have an open channel of elimination for the toxins. (If you do a liver cleanse first and are not able to move toxins through to eliminate quickly, this could lead to re-absorption of toxins causing headaches, nausea, and other problems).

Toxin prevention includes learning how to avoid chemicals and ways we are exposed to them. Many cosmetics include propylene glycol, sodium laurel sulfate, lead, or aluminum. Read labels and look for other products that do not contain these. Products used to wash clothes and dishes also contain many chemicals that are easily absorbed into the skin. Find natural products containing coconut oil or essential oils to use instead.

To get the best results when doing an intestinal cleanse, it is best to avoid or limit certain foods and instead use more beneficial foods. Avoid citrus and berries – these are too acidic. Avoid milk and cheese – these are too congestive for the liver (use soy, almond, or rice milk instead). Avoid coffee – it is too acidic and can upset blood sugar balance and contains oils which can be toxic to the pancreas. Beef, pork, and shellfish are more difficult to digest – eat chicken or fish instead. Eat plenty of fresh and steamed vegetables. Rice is the best carbohydrate to eat. Yams are the best potato to eat. Apples and pears are the best fruits. Drink plenty of water. Use butter, olive oil, or flax seed oil. Avoid sodas, white sugar, and white flour. Gluten in pasta and raised breads is difficult for those with colitis problems. Eat good soups made with broths.

If you get a rash when doing a cleanse, it could mean your body is trying to clear heavy metals. Take more antioxidants (such as **Vitamin C** or **Thai-Go**) to help with this and slow down your cleanse and drink more water. Also support your kidneys with herbal formulas for the kidneys. (Low back pain can be a symptom of metals being released by the kidneys). **MSM** is another supplement that helps release metals. Use bentonite clay for absorbing toxins (such as E-coli). Toxins have a positive charge, bentonite clay has a negative charge, so it absorbs toxins. This is available as **Hydrated Bentonite**. **Clean Start** also contains bentonite clay. Rest and sleep are important to help the body clear toxins. The body cleanses from the head downward. **MSM** helps to clear the lymphatic system and helps the liver to detoxify. **Milk thistle** also helps those exposed to chemicals (such as beauticians or those who work in dry cleaners). **Vita-Lemon** will help remove sluggish material from the gallbladder. **CCA** will help to remove mucous from the body.

A gallbladder cleanse recipe: Take 2 capsules **Cascara sagrada** at bedtime, the next morning, eat a light breakfast of toast or fruit, and then drink apple juice throughout the day consuming 2-4 quarts of juice. Do not eat anything else. You can also take 2 capsules **Cascara sagrada** with breakfast and at noon. At bedtime, take ½ cup extra virgin olive oil and ½ cup fresh squeezed lemon juice, both at room temperature. These can be combined in a blender or taken separately. You can also add 4-6 capsules **Slippery Elm** to this mixture to help prevent nausea. This can be followed by apple juice or grape juice, then go to bed immediately and lay on your right side until falling asleep. In the morning, drink ½ cup warm water and take a water enema. If spasms occur, you may use **Lobelia Essence** rubbed over the gallbladder area. Within 24 hours, you should expel stones, mucous, or sludge through the bowel. This cleanse may be repeated in 14 days. If you need extra support for low blood sugar during this cleanse, you could take 2 or more **Red Beet Root Formula** capsules every 2 hours.

AROMATHERAPY

Aromatherapy is a form of holistic healing. It involves the application or inhaling of pure essential oils to promote physical, emotional, and mental well being. Essential oils are absorbed into the bloodstream within seconds of application on the skin. It is important to obtain quality essential oils since the true oil from the plant or flower will have healing effects. Synthetic oils will not have these effects and are more likely to cause allergic reactions. When using aromatherapy, smell the individual oils. If a particular essential oil smells unpleasant to you at the time, don't use it. Instead, use the ones you find attractive. Safety factors when using essential oils include being careful not to get these in your eyes or mucous membranes.

Lavender is known as a universal oil and is one of the few which can be applied directly on the skin. (It is necessary to use a carrier oil, such as massage oil, to mix with other oils, before applying). The best lavender comes from France. **Lavender** is known for helping with stress and insomnia. It also can be used for burns, including sunburn, as well as skin abrasions or paper cuts. This oil is an ingredient in a recipe for a natural insect repellant along with eucalyptus and thyme. It has also been used to spray on hotel bed sheets to protect against bedbugs. It can be mixed in a spray bottle with purified water and used as a room spray, or as a perfume.

Lemon essential oil has a clean scent and can be used to make a natural household cleaner. This oil will cross the blood-brain barrier (by smelling the oil, it may enhance the effect of other substances). Since this is a citrus oil, never apply this to your skin and go out in the sun – it could cause a sunburn.

Peppermint essential oil is known for helping with digestion. It can help with nausea, just by smelling the oil. A drop or two can be added to water to sip to aid with indigestion. It can be put on feet to help cool off the body and ease tired feet. This oil is an ingredient in a recipe for Hot Flash Spray. The best peppermint comes from Oregon.

Bergamot essential oil is known for helping with depression and anxiety. Add 3-10 drops to a bath for a relaxing soak. The best bergamot comes from Italy where it grows as a non-edible fruit. This also is a citrus oil, so be careful about going in the sun after using it.

Pink Grapefruit essential oil is uplifting and helps the mood. It has also been used to reduce cellulite on the skin by mixing with a carrier oil and applying. This is another citrus oil.

Red Mandarin essential oil has been used to help with acid reflux – mix with a carrier oil and apply over area of upper chest. It is also a citrus oil that originates from Italy.

Rose essential oil is one of the most expensive oils. The best rose oil comes from Bulgaria. It takes 5000 pounds of rose petals to equal 1 pound of essential oil. Rose has been known to be used for grief and bereavement, for heart palpitations, for menopausal concerns, and for cosmetic uses.

Roman Chamomile essential oil is an antispasmodic and helps against inflammation. This oil comes from France. It has been used with a carrier oil to rub on the abdomen for cases of colitis, irritable bowel problems, and any spasms in the intestines.

Eucalyptus essential oil is antifungal and has been used for respiratory problems. It has helped respiratory problems by use of a diffuser in a room or by putting a few drops in a bowl of hot water and inhaling the steam. This oil comes from Spain.

Tea Tree oil has a very distinctive smell and originates from Australia. It has been used for skin and nail infections and for oral care. A few drops can be added to a foot basin for a foot soak to help with toenail fungus. This oil can be applied directly on the skin for wounds or insect bites, but may cause a burning sensation.

Frankincense essential oil is known for use as incense in church. It has been known to aid in meditation. It also can help the respiratory system in cases of asthma. Inhaling the scent helps with deep breathing. It comes from Somalia.